LIVING WITH MENOPAUSE

(Defy Age With Confidence And Grace)

'Denike Owolabi

Living With Menopause

Ordering Details

To place orders or for details of discounts for bulk purchases by organizations or groups either for support, gift, training packages, fundraising, or any other educational purposes, send an email to denikeowolabi65@gmail.com.

Table of Contents

DEDICATION

This book holds a deep gratitude for someone truly special. In memory of the late Pst Mrs Sarah Oluwaseun Ojeme, whose unwavering support, including financial assistance for radio broadcasts, made this book possible. Her heart was as precious as gold, and I miss her dearly.

Every page of this book is touched by her kindness and encouragement. Though she may not be physically present, her legacy of goodness and generosity lives on. I miss the sound of her laughter and the warmth of her spirit, but her impact remains strong.

This book is dedicated to you, Pst (Mrs) Sarah Oluwaseun Ojeme.

With heartfelt gratitude and enduring love,

'Denike Owolabi

FOREWORD

This is not just a book, but a literary work that is informative, educative, academic, erudite and transformative.

It is a manual that will bring succour to many hurting women going through the inevitable experience of menopause.

Mrs Owolabi is not writing from only a professional perspective but from a personal existential position of personal experience by someone with a first hand knowledge of menopause.

I therefore recommend this book, not just for women, but also for their husbands and family members.

In a time when we seem to have so much information but less education, this is a timely book. May you find fulfilment and resolutions from this book.

Abraham Olufemi Ojeme,
Founder/CEO, Builders Forum Global Inc.

ACKNOWLEDGEMENTS

Putting the information contained in this book together, has been a journey of exploration, understanding, and collaboration, and I am deeply grateful to the individuals who have played an instrumental role in bringing this work to fruition.

First and foremost, I extend my heartfelt gratitude to the countless women who shared their stories, experiences, and wisdom on the subject of menopause. Your openness and resilience have enriched the pages of this book and contributed to a more comprehensive understanding of this important life transition.

I am indebted to my family for their unwavering support and encouragement throughout the writing process. Your patience, understanding, and belief in the significance of this project have been a source of strength. My daughter, Timi, thank you for coming up with the story of Alice and writing the lyrics of the

Living With Menopause soundtrack.

To the experts and professionals in the fields of women's health, who generously shared their insights, thank you for contributing your expertise to enhance the accuracy and depth of the content.

I am especially grateful to Matrons Pat Odia, Priscilla Echabor and Philomena Moriah for their support when "Living With Menopause" was aired on radio.

My director, Iroro Agarry and editor, Paul Kpologri, thank you.

Dcns Titilayo Adesoji and Dcns Evelyn Olore Imokhe, I can't forget your financial contribution to this project. Thank you.

To Mrs Grace Olumayowa Aideloje, I say thank you, for patiently proofreading and editing this work at short notice. My friend and sister, Mrs Oyeyemi Jimi-Salami, thank you for your honest review when you read the manuscript.

Lastly, to the readers - thank you for

embarking on this journey with me. It is my sincere hope that the information within these pages serves as a source of empowerment, understanding, and connection for women navigating the profound and transformative phase of menopause.

With gratitude, 'Denike Owolabi

INTRODUCTION

The Story of Alice

Alice was young and beautiful, full of life and ready to live that life to the fullest. When her husband first saw her, he said she was as bright as the "Sunshine".

Alice's life was filled with love, joy, and dreams of a glorious future. Her husband admired and loved her passionately and together, they tirelessly nurtured their beautiful family, raising their children with care and pursuing successful careers. You can say Alice had it together, what a Joy!!!

Her vibrant spirit and unwavering determination shaped her life, but just when she thought she was close to harvesting seeds sown, IT HAPPENED!!!

What happened?

Life took an unexpected turn.

Unexpected challenges came knocking and she found herself facing a journey she never anticipated.

Symptoms began to surface. Irregular menstrual periods, leaving her unsure and concerned about her own body.

Sometimes, it'd be so scanty and at other times, it would be so heavy that she would be afraid of losing all the blood in her body.

Then came this heat from her chest up that she just couldn't explain. It would leave her drenched in her own sweat to the point where she would feel like taking of her clothes in the midst of people.

Palpitations and localized headaches that would make you forget your name became her constant companions, threatening to engulf her.

So, Alice started consulting from one hospital to another, symptoms were treated but they kept coming back. Lasting relief remained elusive.

As is common in our African culture, well-meaning friends and relatives suggested alternative remedies. Confused in and really seeking solutions, Alice embarked on another journey. Off she went from one "baba" to another, to prayer houses, to fake prophets, to spiritualists and of course, this came with enough harvest of visions about enemies and witches.

As you would expect, precious relationships were destroyed in the process as some persons in her life were labeled as being behind her ordeal.

Unfortunately, despite all her efforts, the sacrifices and letting go of her sophistication (as it were), hoping to find relief, the symptoms persisted, and her hope began to wane.

Alice's pursuit of healing had led her down a path of uncertainty, vulnerability and financial strain. As her bank balance depleted, she wondered if she would ever live to see the fruit of her labor in her husband's and children's lives.

Alice, the beauty, once nicknamed 'SUNSHINE WOMAN' by her husband, had become ashadow of herself.

Alice's story is the story of many African women who are ignorant of or have very little knowledge of the different seasons of a woman's life.

Alice came to the season of menopause and she didn't know it. Not that she had not heard the word 'menopause' before, but she never knew what she should expect approaching it and while in it.

But dear reader, don't get scared; there is hope in the midst of darkness. Every woman can navigate through the different seasons of life, including menopause, in a healthy and positive way with grace and knowledge. It's about understanding that menopause is a part of the natural aging process for every woman who will live long. It is about understanding the changes and sometimes challenges that come with it and embracing them without feeling overwhelmed.

What is more, each woman's experience with menopause is unique, just like each woman's experience in pregnancy. Not all women go through serious symptoms or difficulty in menopause like Alice; some breeze through it.

This book, 'Living with Menopause,' aims to enlighten women on their journey through menopause and empower them to navigate this season of life with confidence, grace and knowledge. From understanding the physical changes, to managing emotions, we will provide information to help you embrace this phase of life confidently.

This is 2023, I am in my late fifties now and of course in my post menopause years. It's been quite an 'interesting experience' in which knowledge has played a significant role.

I invite you to join me on this journey. Let's debunk myths, share experiences, and create a community of support and understanding.

Together, we will navigate through menopause, appreciating the beauty of every season in life.

AGING IS NOT DYING

THE CALL

There comes a time in a woman's life when a profound and transformative change takes place. It is a phase that has been whispered about in hushed tones, steeped in misconceptions and misinformation. Yet, it is a journey that every woman will embark upon: the journey of menopause.

This is a call to all African women, a call to embrace menopause as a natural and empowering phase of life. It is a call to get educated on this transformative experience, to replace fear and uncertainty with knowledge and understanding.

It is time to shine a light on this journey, to celebrate the wisdom, strength, and beauty that come with it. Together, we will explore the physical changes, the emotional rollercoaster, and the unique challenges faced by African women.

I call on you to embark on a voyage of discovery on the pages of this book and learn about the intricacies of our bodies, the complexities of our emotions, and the power of our resilience through this significant phase of life.

Let us step into the light, shedding the culture of silence and embracing menopause as a catalyst for growth, transformation, and a newfound sense of purpose. Together, we will navigate the challenges and embrace the beauty that lies within the embrace of menopause.

AGING IS NOT DYING

Spark Of Passion

The spark for my passion in the subject of menopause ignited from observations and genuine concern.

During my time as a practice manager at a hospital in my twenties, I began to notice common complaints among women of a particular age group. This trend extended beyond just the patients; it resonated among relatives, neighbors, church members, acquaintances, and beyond. My innate love for knowledge and thirst for information drove me to investigate further, seeking to uncover the underlying reasons. My exploration eventually led me to the subject of menopause.

While encountering women seeking medical attention for their symptoms was not unusual, it was however sad to discover that many women entering this phase lacked adequate information. As a result, they often interpreted the symptoms of menopause as spiritual afflictions or a form of malevolence from others.

Moreover, I encountered a few women who were still on their journey to conceive when they found themselves on the cusp of menopause. They faced confusion, mistaking irregular menstruation for pregnancy or pregnancy loss without proper testing. My heart especially goes out to these women.

Let me emphasize that I firmly believe in

miracles, and with God, all things are possible. Regardless of menopause or your age, God's ability to bless you with your own biological children remains unaffected.

With that being said, it remains of utmost importance that women in this particular phase possess a deep understanding of what menopause entails to shield themselves from emotional instability and vulnerability.

Now, let's delve into the meaning of Menopause.

Chapter 1

What Is Menopause?

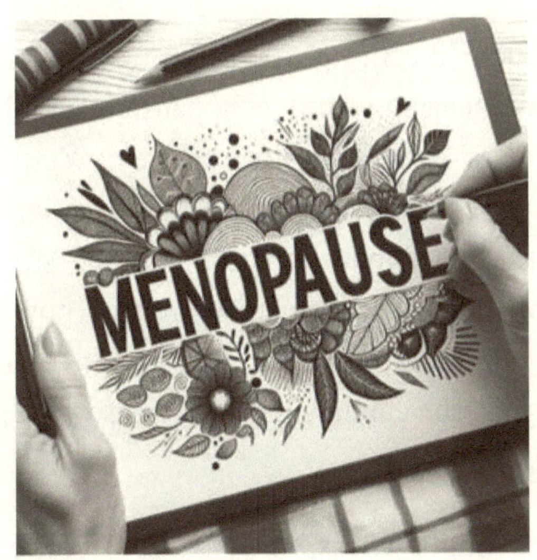
image created with Microsoft Bing AI Image Creator

In the last pages, I provided an insightful introduction to the subject of Menopause. I encourage you not to rush over it, as it offers valuable information.

What Is Menopause?

MENOPAUSE is a natural and inevitable process that accompanies the journey of aging. As long as a woman desires and embraces the gift of longevity—a hope cherished by us all—she will undoubtedly go through the path of menopause and its transitional shifts.

Much like the passage through puberty or the childbearing years, menopause is an integral part of a woman's life journey. Yet, it is imperative to emphasize that this transition need not drive a woman crazy or take the sunshine out of her life. Armed with the power of knowledge and equipped with effective coping strategies, she can navigate this phase with grace and resilience.

In simple terms, menopause signifies the closure of a woman's menstrual cycles, signaling the end of her reproductive era. This is of course talking about natural menopause, one that is notinduced by medical interventions.

Natural menopause is not sudden; it unfolds gradually and manifests in three distinct stages.

1. Peri-Menopause - This pivotal phase can commence around 8 to 10 years before the onset of menopause. Typically, it kicks off in a woman's forties and persists until menopause is achieved.

During peri-menopause, a gradual reduction in estrogen production by the ovaries takes place. Menstruation still occurs at this juncture, and the woman can still get pregnant.

It's important to note that the decline in estrogen intensifies or accelerates during the last one to two years of peri-menopause. This acceleration can trigger various symptoms.

I have observed that it is this period that often hosts a spectrum of dramas related to menopausal symptoms that make some women vulnerable as exemplified in the story of Alice.

2. Menopause - This phase marks a significant milestone: the complete cessation of menstrual periods. It's characterized by the ovaries stopping the release of eggs and producing significantly less estrogen.

3. Post Menopause - This term refers to the period following an entire year without a menstrual period, equating 12 consecutive months of no menstruation.

For many women who experienced challenging menopausal symptoms, this stage often brings some relief but also ushers in a predisposition to some specific health challenges. Examples include, osteoporosis and heart problems, which can be effectively managed with lifestyle changes and medical interventions."

These distinct phases of the menopausal journey encompass various changes, symptoms, and adaptations. It's crucial to understand and navigate each stage with grace and awareness, fostering an environment of self-care and understanding.

What is the normal age of menopause and how is it diagnosed? This will be the focus in the next chapter.

To conclude, let's reflect on the multifaceted journey of a woman's life - a journey that spans from the tender phase of puberty to the nurturing years of motherhood and child-rearing, and ultimately leads to the significant phase of menopause and post menopause.

Each of these seasons holds its own significance, as they usher in changes that are often accompanied by new challenges.

Embracing the uniqueness of each phase, and recognizing that challenges are inherent to change, every woman has the potential to navigate through these life stages naturally, healthily, and positively.

Please know this and know it well, menopause is simply one of the natural seasons in a woman's life; it's not a disease or an anomaly.

And always remember, aging is not synonymous with dying. Aging Is Not Dying!

Chapter 2

Understanding The Onset, Influences, and Diagnosis of Menopause.

This chapter will help you to understand when menopause starts, what affects the timing and how it is diagnosed.

It's important to know that menopause is different for everyone. The way you experience it can be very unique. Some women might go through it without many problems, while others might have more noticeable changes in their body and feelings. It's good to remember that menopause is a natural part of the aging process of a woman and not a sickness or an anomaly.

By understanding the different stages of

menopause, you can better understand what is happening in your body and thus eliminate fears, confusion and agitations. This knowledge can also help you make smart choices about your health and find the right help and information during your menopause journey.

You are not alone – many women have gone through or are going through menopause, and together we can handle it gracefully and with confidence.

When Does Menopause Start?

On average, menopause starts around age 51. But it's important to know that the timing can be different for each person. Some women might start menopause a bit earlier, usually in their late 40s or early 50s, while others might experience it later, like in their mid-50s or even early 60s. A few factors can influence when menopause happens. Let's look at some of these things:

1. Genes

Your genes, the things you inherit from

your family, can play a big part in when you start menopause. If your mother or other female family members went through menopause earlier or later, you might follow a similar pattern. But it is important to know that genes are not the only thing that matters, and sometimes things can be different.

2. Lifestyle and Health

Certain things you do and your health can also affect when menopause happens. For example,

- Smoking: Studies show that smoking can make menopause start earlier. Smoking is linked to many health problems and can also make your ovaries stop working sooner.

- Body Weight: Women who have a lower body weight might start menopause earlier than those who weigh more.

- Health Issues and Treatments: Some medical conditions and treatments, like having surgery on your ovaries, going through chemotherapy, or getting radiation, can affect when menopausestarts.

- Ethnic Background: Research suggests that your ethnic background can also play a role. For example, studies show that African American and Hispanic women might start menopause a bit earlier than women from other backgrounds.

3. Your History:

Things like when you first got your period and how many times you have been pregnant can also influence when menopause happens. Women who started their periods early or had fewer pregnancies might start menopause earlier.

Remember, even though these things can give us some clues, when menopause happens can still be different for everyone. It's a mix of genes, lifestyle, and other things.

Understanding when menopause usually starts and what can affect when it happens can help you know more about your own experience. Face it with kindness toward yourself and seek for support and resources that can help you personally.

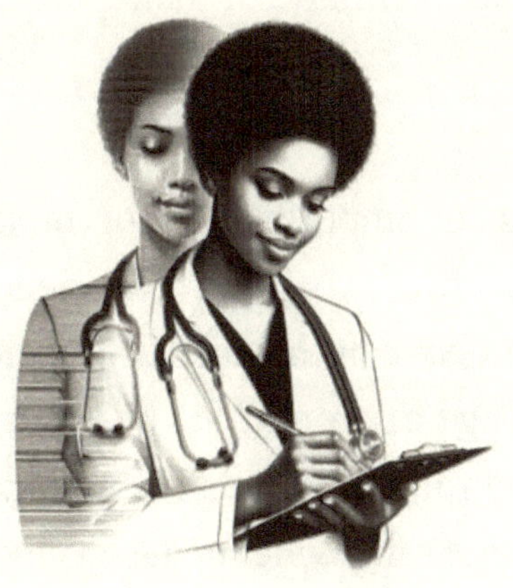

image created with Microsoft Bing AI Image Creator

How Menopause Is Diagnosed

Diagnosing menopause involves a combination of clinical assessment, symptoms evaluation, and sometimes laboratory tests.

1. Clinical Assessment

This is done by a doctor discussing the woman's medical history, including menstrual patterns and any symptoms she may be experiencing. Information about the frequency and duration of periods, as well as the presence of symptoms like hot flashes, night sweats, mood changes, and vaginal dryness, helps in assessing the likelihood of menopause.

2. Age

This is an important factor in diagnosing menopause. Most women experience natural menopause between the ages of 45 and 55, with an average age of around 51. If a woman has not had a period for 12 consecutive months and is in the typical age range, menopause is likely.

3. Blood Tests

These can be done to measure hormone levels, specifically FSH (Follicle-Stimulating Hormone) and Estrogen. FSH is a hormone released by the pituitary gland that stimulates the ovaries to produce estrogen and develop eggs. As a woman's ovarian function decreases during menopause, the pituitary gland produces more FSH to stimulate the ovaries. Elevated FSH levels, along with decreased estrogen levels, are often indicative of menopause.

4. Hormone Levels

While FSH levels increase during menopause, Estrogen levels decrease. Estrogen is a key reproductive hormone responsible for regulating the menstrual cycle and maintaining various bodily functions in a woman. A significant drop in estrogen levels contributes to many of the symptoms associated with menopause.

5. Other Tests

In some cases, additional tests like thyroid function tests or prolactin levels may be done to rule out other conditions that could be causing symptoms similar to those of menopause.

In summary, diagnosing menopause involves considering a combination of factors, including a woman's age, symptoms, and hormone levels. Consulting a healthcare professional is advised to ensure an accurate diagnosis and appropriate management of symptoms.

In conclusion, gaining a comprehensive

understanding of when menopause starts, the factors influencing its timing, and the diagnostic methods involved empowers the woman to navigate this natural life transition with confidence and knowledge.

Aging Is Not Dying!

A Word For Those Trying to Conceive

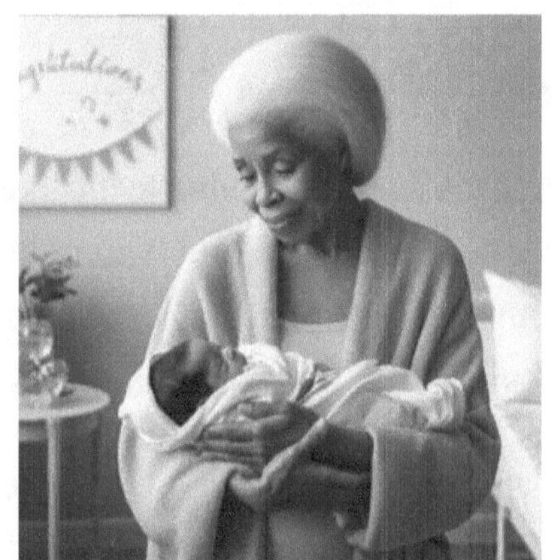

image created with Microsoft Bing AI Image Creator

If you are still on the journey of fruitfulness, with the path to motherhood veiled in uncertainty, and have found yourself standing at the doorstep of menopause, let me share a truth with you – the promises of God regarding fruitfulness do not expire with menopause.

The pages of history and the Bible are adorned with countless stories of miraculous births to women who, against all odds, believed in the divine promise.

Hannah's tears and longing turned into the laughter of Samuel, and Elizabeth's years of waiting birthed the heralding cry of John the Baptist. Sarah's testimony is an everlasting testimonial.

These stories are not just tales of the past; they are living testimonies, assuring us that miracles happen.

Menopause may be an undeniable natural reality, but with unwavering faith, it doesn't have the final say in your journey to motherhood. There are numerous accounts of women, post-menopause in contemporary times, experiencing the joy of miracle babies even after menopause tried to say "it was too late"– a testament to the enduring power of faith.

I urge you to look beyond the visible, into the realm of the miraculous.

So, anytime you find yourself in the shadow

of doubt or discouragement, remember this, miracles are not confined to the pages of the Holy Book, they are inscribed in the narratives of our contemporary lives as well. The miracle you believe in is the next one in line.

For every Sarah, there's a miracle named Isaac. For every Elizabeth, there's a miracle named John. Your name, too, can be elegantly printed in the scroll of miracles.

Hold on to your dreams, your prayers, and your faith. The one who is full of mercy, hears the quiet whispers of your heart, and sees your tear-stained prayers. You are not alone.

Do not let menopause drown out the hope inside you, hold on to your faith, for it's a force that can turn the page of impossibility into a chapter of miracles. Do not be dismayed or discouraged, for your story is still unfolding, God is not finished with you, and the Author of miracles is not finished writing.

Know this deep in your heart – miracles happen, and they can happen for you too. I BELIEVE IN MIRACLES!

Chapter 3

Hormonal Changes in Menopause

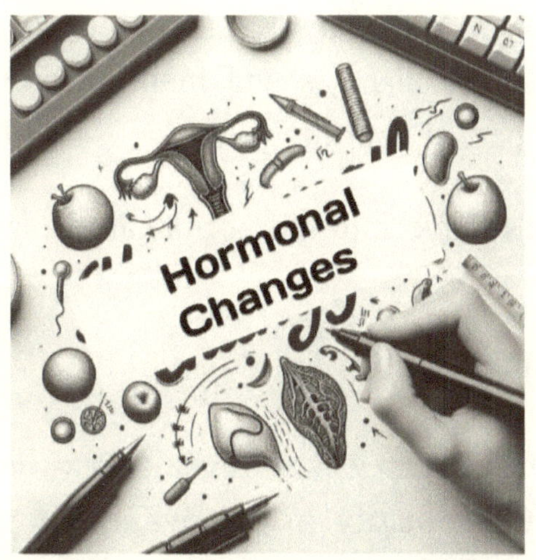

image created with Microsoft Bing AI Image Creator

Menopause is marked by significant hormonal changes in a woman's body. The primary hormones affected during this transition are Estrogen and Progesterone, which play crucial roles in the menstrual cycle and reproductive processes. Understanding these hormonal changes can provide valuable insights into the symptoms and effects experienced during menopause.

In other words, understanding what is happening in your body is the first step to taking good care of yourself during menopause and eliminating panic. Just know that you are not alone, and many resources can help you handle these changes and make menopause a natural part of your life's story.

Let's delve into the hormonal changes that occur:

1. Estrogen

Estrogen is a key female sex hormone produced primarily in the ovaries. It plays a vital role in regulating the menstrual cycle and supporting reproductive health. During menopause, the production of estrogen gradually declines. However, the decline is not linear and can fluctuate, leading to hormonal imbalances and irregular menstrual cycles during perimenopause.

Lower estrogen levels can contribute to various physical and emotional symptoms commonly linked with menopause. They include hot flashes (when you suddenly feel very hot and sweaty), night sweats, vaginal dryness, changes in skin elasticity, and mood swings. Estrogen also playsa role in maintaining bone density, so decreased levels can increase the risk of osteoporosis or bone density loss. "

2. Progesterone

Progesterone is another important hormone involved in the menstrual cycle and pregnancy. It works in conjunction with estrogen to regulate the buildup and shedding of the uterine lining. During perimenopause, progesterone levels may become irregular. This can make your periods act strangely – they might be heavier or lighter than usual.

3. Follicle-Stimulating Hormone (FSH)

When your ovaries start making less

estrogen, your brain says, "Hey, make more!" This brain message comes as a hormone called FSH. It tells your ovaries to work harder.

Elevated FSH levels during menopause are often responsible for irregular periods and can contribute to other symptoms such as mood changes or fluctuations and sleep disturbances (inability to fall asleep and stay asleep as you desire).

4. Luteinizing Hormone (LH)

This is closely associated with the menstrual cycle and ovulation. During perimenopause, LH levels may become more erratic. LH levels surge right before ovulation, and this surge can become more unpredictable during the menopause transition. This hormonal imbalance can lead to irregular menstrual cycles and contribute to symptoms such as hot flashes.

These hormonal fluctuations can vary from woman to woman, resulting in a wide range of experiences during menopause. It's important to remember that how you experience menopause that is, how your body responds to the effects of hormonal changes during menopause is individual and can be influenced by various factors such as genetics, overall health, and lifestyle.

If you are experiencing significant challenges or discomfort due to hormonal changes during menopause, it's advisable to consult with a healthcare professional. They can provide guidance and discuss potential treatment options, to manage symptoms and promote overall well-being during this transformative phase.

In conclusion, understanding the hormonal changes that occur during menopause can empower you to make informed decisions or smart choices about your health and seek appropriate support when needed.

AGING IS NOT DYING!

Chapter 4

Understanding Common Physical Symptoms Of Menopause

Menopause brings about a range of physical symptoms that can vary in intensity and duration for each individual. While not all women will experience every symptom, being aware of the common physical changes can help you recognize, and manage them effectively as well as rule out fear and panic.

Let's explore some of the most frequently encountered physical symptoms during menopause:

1. Irregular Menstrual Cycles:

As you approach menopause, that is at peri-menopause, your menstrual cycles may become irregular. You may experience changes in the frequency, duration, and flow of your periods. Some women may have shorter, lighter periods, while others may have longer, heavier ones. It's important to note that irregular bleeding should always be discussed with a healthcare professional to rule out other potential causes.

2. Hot Flashes and Night Sweats:

Hot flashes are perhaps the most well-known symptom of menopause. They are characterized by a sudden sensation of heat that spreads throughout the body, often accompanied by flushing of the face and excessive sweating. Night sweats are similar but occur specifically during sleep, leading to drenched nightclothes and disrupted sleep patterns.

3. Vaginal Dryness and Changes in Sexual Health:

Decreased estrogen levels can cause

changes in the vaginal tissues, leading to vaginal dryness, itching, and discomfort during sexual intercourse. These changes may affect sexual desire and arousal. Fortunately, there are various lubricants and moisturizers available to alleviate vaginal dryness and enhance comfort.

4. Sleep Disturbances:

Menopause can disrupt sleep patterns, making it difficult to fall asleep or stay asleep throughout the night.

Night-time hot flashes and night sweats can contribute to sleep disturbances. Poor sleep quality can lead to daytime fatigue, mood changes, and reduced overall well-being.

Exercising for at least fifteen minutes at night has been a great help to me in overcoming this. Find what works for you naturally to avoid addiction to sleeping pills and potential side effects.

5. Changes in Skin and Hair:

Fluctuating hormone levels can affect the skin and hair. Some women may experience dryness, itchiness, and thinning of the skin. Additionally, hair may become drier, thinner, or more prone to breakage. Adapting skincare and hair care routines can help mitigate these effects.

6. Changes in Body Composition and Weight:

During menopause, some women may notice changes in body composition, including an increase in abdominal fat and a loss of muscle mass. These changes can impact body shape and weight distribution. Maintaining a healthy lifestyle, including regular exercise and a balanced diet, can help manage weight and support overall well-being.

7. Bone Health:

Estrogen plays a crucial role in maintaining bone density. With decreasing estrogen levels during menopause, women become more susceptible to bone loss and osteoporosis. Ensuring an adequate intake of calcium and vitamin D (under the guidance of your doctor), along with weight-bearing exercises, can help support bone health.

Now you know why some older women complain of knee pains, walk the way they do and at times support the hips and waist with their hands.

It's important to remember that while these physical symptoms can be challenging, they are a normal part of the menopause transition and are due to decreasing or fluctuating hormones associated with menopause.

If you find that these symptoms significantly impact your quality of life, don't hesitate to seek support from healthcare professionals. They can provide guidance and discuss potential treatment options tailored to your specific needs.

Remember, every woman's menopause experience is unique. By staying informed and proactive, you can better manage the physical symptoms of menopause and prioritize your overall health and well-being.

Aging Is Not Dying!

Chapter 5

Exploring Emotional And Psychological Changes During Menopause

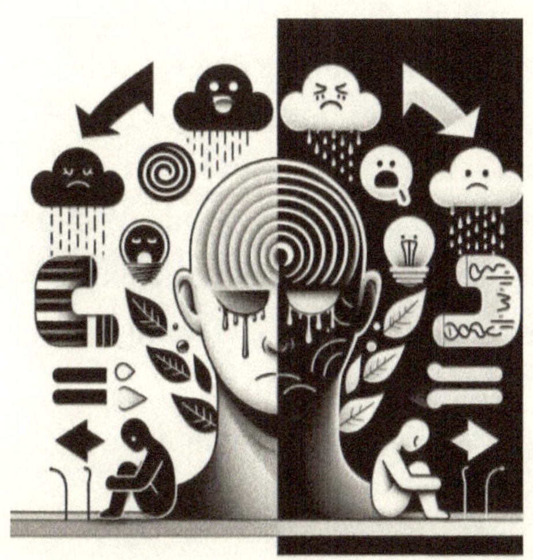

image created with Microsoft Bing AI Image Creator

Menopause not only brings physical changes but also impacts emotional and psychological well-being.

The fluctuating hormone levels and life transitions associated with this phase can contribute to various emotional symptoms (rollercoaster of emotions). Understanding and acknowledging these changes can help you navigate them with greater ease.

Let's delve into the emotional and psychological aspects of menopause: Mood Swings:

Hormonal fluctuations during menopause can lead to mood swings, characterized by rapid and

intense changes in mood. You may find yourself experiencing heightened irritability, sadness, anxiety, or feelings of being overwhelmed. One moment, you may be giggling with friends, and the next, you feel like snapping.

These mood swings can sometimes be challenging to manage, but they are a common part of the menopause journey. You may find solace in taking deep breaths at such times.

Fatigue and Lack of Energy:

Many women going through menopause report increased feelings of fatigue and a general lack of energy. Hormonal changes, sleep disturbances, and the physical symptoms associated with menopause can all contribute to this sense of tiredness. It's important to prioritize self-care, including getting enough rest and engaging in activities that recharge your energy levels.

Anxiety and Restlessness:

Menopause can bring about feelings of anxiety and restlessness. You may experience a heightened sense of worry, nervousness, or unease. These emotional changes can be attributed to both hormonal fluctuations and the psychological impact of adjusting to life transitions that often coincide with menopause.

While menopause itself does not cause clinical depression, some women may experience feelings of sadness or depression during this phase.

If you find that your feelings of depression persist or interfere with your daily life, it's essential to seek professional support.

I found myself many times during my transition suddenly feeling very sad, to the point where I just wanted to cry. I know I am not alone, neither are you. At such a times, do something thatmakes you happy.

Memory Issues and Cognitive Changes:

Some women may notice changes in memory, concentration, and cognitive function during menopause. These changes are often referred to as "menopause brain fog."

Have you ever entered a room only to forget what you came there for, forget where you left your keys or blank out during meetings?

While the exact cause is not fully

understood, hormonal fluctuations and sleep disturbances may contribute to these cognitive symptoms. Engaging in mental exercises (e.g., puzzles, brain teasers), maintaining a healthy lifestyle, and managing stress can help support cognitive function.

Self-esteem and Body Image:

Menopause can sometimes affect a woman's self-esteem and body image. The physical changes that occur, such as weight fluctuations, changes in skin, and hair thinning, can impact how women perceive themselves. It's important to remember that beauty and worthiness are not defined by physical appearance alone.

My hair was once thick and very full and I felt very proud combing it in a salon to the admiration of all present, however, it has since become a 'private part' for me.

If you are noticing some extra curves and thinner hair, it may be hard but it is important at this time to nurture a positive self-image, reduce calorie in-take and increase physical activities like aerobics & strength training exercises.

Practice self-compassion and remind yourself daily that you are beautiful and a strong woman, inside and out.

It's crucial to recognize that emotional and psychological changes during menopause are valid and should be addressed. If you find that these symptoms significantly impact your daily life or overall well-being, consider reaching out to a healthcare professional or mental health specialist. They can provide guidance, support, and potential treatment options tailored to your specific needs.

Remember, you are not alone in navigating the emotional aspects of menopause. Connecting with supportive friends, family, or participating in support groups and feeding yourself with relevant information can offer comfort and understanding.

Embrace self-care practices, engage in activities that bring you joy, and prioritize your emotional well-being throughout this transformative phase.

In the next chapter, I will bring you some uncommon symptoms of menopause you should be aware of to eliminate fear and panic.

Aging Is Not Dying!

Chapter 6

Exploring Some Uncommon Symptoms of Menopause

Menopause, a natural phase in a woman's life, brings about various changes due to shifts in hormone levels. While some women breeze through menopause, others encounter unique and uncommon symptoms that can be bewildering. It is essential to understand these symptoms as they may affect your quality of life.

Here, we delve into some of the lesser-known menopausal symptoms:

1. Formication: The Creeping Sensation:

Formication is a peculiar sensation characterized by the feeling of tiny insects crawling under your skin. This sensation can be rather unpleasant and irritating, often leading to bouts of itching and scratching, day or night, on various parts of your body.

This unusual symptom is often linked to low estrogen levels, a hallmark of menopause. As estrogen levels decline, so does the production of collagen, a protein crucial for maintaining healthy skin. Estrogen typically stimulates collagen production. Consequently, this hormonal shift can result in thinner and drier skin, making it more prone to itching. Additionally, you might become more sensitive to soaps and detergents during this phase.

Managing formication can usually be self-directed, for instance, through the use of moisturizers to soothe the skin.

However, if this symptom becomes bothersome or persistent, it's advisable to consult a medical professional. They can offer guidance on alternative self-care remedies or potentially refer you to a dermatologist for specialized advice.

I have witnessed this particular symptom causing emotional, mental, and psychological challenges for some women. When it comes to handling menopause, knowledge plays a crucial role.

2. Mouth Problems or Oral Changes:

The drop in estrogen during menopause can impact your oral health. This may manifest as burning tongue, gum disease, or persistent dry mouth. These symptoms can affect your sense of taste, cause discomfort, and even lead to gum problems and tooth decay. Good dental hygiene, hydration, and avoiding certain substances can help alleviate these issues.

3. Body Odours:

Menopausal changes like hot flashes and shifts in vaginal mucus can lead to body odours. These changes can alter the balance of microorganisms in your body, affecting the smell of sweat and vaginal discharge.

However, during menopause, some women might experience an increased sense of smell.

This means that the odours you notice might not be detectable by others!

4. **Tinnitus:** Ringing in the Ears:

Tinnitus, often referred to as the perception of 'ringing in your ears,' is a condition where you hear sounds that are not originating from external sources. While tinnitus is typically not a cause for immediate concern, it can range from a minor annoyance to something profoundly distressing.

Fluctuations in hormone levels in menopause can influence the auditory system, leading to these sounds, particularly during the perimenopausal and menopausal stages.

Dealing with tinnitus may involve several self-care strategies, including:

- Regular Exercise: Engaging in physical activity can help improve blood circulation, which may alleviate tinnitus symptoms.

- Stress Management: Stress can exacerbate tinnitus. Practicing stress-reduction techniques may provide relief.

- Noise Avoidance: Loud noises can worsen tinnitus. Be mindful of your environment and protect your ears when exposed to loud sounds.

- Adequate Rest: Fatigue can intensify tinnitus. Ensure you are getting enough sleep to minimize its impact.

It is essential to remember that tinnitus can have various causes, and its management may differ from person to person. If tinnitus persists or worsens, consulting a healthcare professional is advisable to rule out any underlying issues and explore potential treatments or therapies.

5. Electric Shocks:

Occasional jolts of pain, like electric shocks, may occur before or during hot flashes. These sensations are thought to result from misfiring neurons in the nervous system due to hormonal changes.

6\. Cold Flushes:

While hot flushes are widely recognized as a common menopausal symptom, cold flushes, or sudden chills, can also affect some women during this phase of life. These cold episodes may occur independently or in conjunction with hot flushes, creating a unique menopausal experience.

Cold flushes typically involve a sudden sensation of feeling chilled. Although they tend to be of short duration, often lasting only a few minutes, they can disrupt sleep patterns and leave you feeling fatigued in the morning.

The underlying cause of cold flushes can be attributed to hormonal fluctuations that impact the hypothalamus, the brain's temperature regulator. This disruption in temperature regulation can lead to these chilly episodes. Interestingly, some women experience chills immediately following a hot flush as their body strives to regain temperature equilibrium.

If you find that your menopausal chills tend to occur after a hot flush, there are lifestyle adjustments you can make to potentially alleviate them. It's advisable to avoid triggers like alcohol, caffeine, and spicy foods, which have the potential to induce hot flushes. By managing these factors, you may experience fewer cold flushes and a more comfortable menopausal journey.

7. Tingling or Numbness: Tingling or numbness, known as paresthesia, can affect various body parts, such as the hands, feet, arms, and legs. As estrogen levels decline, the central nervous system may be affected, leading to these sensations. To alleviate them, maintain a healthy lifestyle and consult a doctor if they persist or worsen.

These lesser-known menopausal symptoms can accompany the more common ones. If you experience these symptoms, know that you are not alone, and there is no need to fear.

However, if you are concerned or the symptoms persist or worsen, consult your healthcare practitioner for guidance and support on managing menopause effectively.

Knowledge empowers women to recognize, manage, and embrace both the common and less typical aspects of this life transition. By shedding light on the uncommon symptoms and experiences, we can dispel the anxieties that can accompany menopause and replace them with informed decision-making and a sense of empowerment.

Therefore, in the realm of menopause, information plays an indispensable role, offering a guiding light through what can be an emotionally and physically challenging but ultimately liberating phase in a woman's life.

Aging Is Not Dying!

The Journey of Menopause
(My Experience)

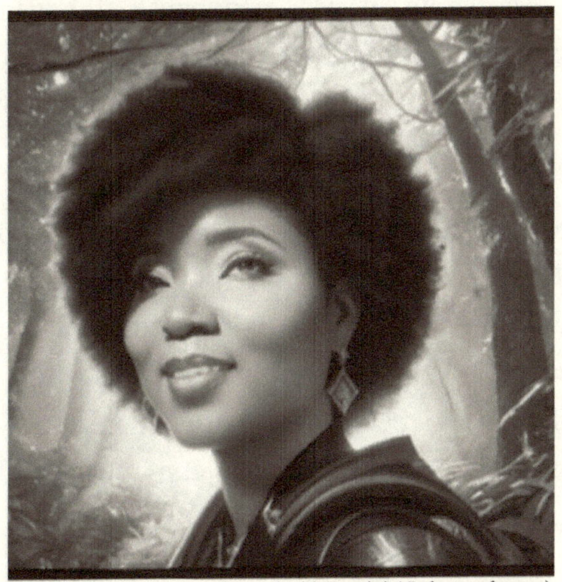

'Denike Owolabi (image enhanced with Remini AI photo enhancer)

I had always looked forward to the phase of life known as menopause. Of course, like many other women, for years, I had dealt with the challenges of menstruation and family planning, and I was ready for a change. With the knowledge I had consciously sought out, I was prepared (or so I thought) to face whatever set of unique experiences and challenges this journey could bring with positivity, grace and understanding.

As I entered peri-menopause, I began to experience irregular menstrual periods, localized headaches, and fainting episodes.

The latter, was a strange sensation, as if the ground beneath me was unsteady and I could fall at any moment. These episodes were accompanied by heart palpitations that would leave me feeling scared and anxious. I knew I had to seek medical help to understand what was happening to my body and rule out other causes apart from menopause.

After undergoing various tests, no abnormalities were found. It was then that I realized these symptoms were part of the menopause journey for me. Armed with this knowledge, I began to cope with the fainting episodes and heart palpitations in a different way. While the physical sensations were still unsettling, I found solace in knowing that they were a natural part of this phase of life for me, as every woman's experience is unique.

For the fainting episodes, I learned to take care of myself by ensuring I stayed hydrated and well-rested. I also made sure to keep a close eye on my blood sugar levels, as low blood sugar could trigger these episodes. Additionally, I found comfort in knowing that these episodes weretemporary and would eventually pass.

As for the heart palpitations, I sought medical help as well and was prescribed medication to help manage them. Taking the prescribed medication provided some relief, although it took time for my body to adjust it. It was a challenging period, but I remained hopeful that these symptoms would subside as I progressed further into menopause.

Despite having knowledge about menopause and its associated symptoms, actually going through it was a different experience altogether. The physical symptoms I experienced were sometimes scary, even though I understood their connection to menopause. It was a reminder that every individual's journey through menopause is unique and can bring unexpected challenges.

During this phase,

- I found support and resources online. I sought out information to educate myself further on the topic, which helped me better understand what was happening to my body as I progress in the journey. Having this knowledge prevented me from associating the symptoms with malevolence or other unrelated causes. It gave me a sense of empowerment and allowed me to approach the journey with a more positive mindset.

- I learned to embrace the journey of menopause as a natural part of aging, a universal experience, transcending cultural boundaries.

- I discovered the importance of self-care, both physically and emotionally. I made sure to prioritize my well-being by engaging in activities that brought me joy and relaxation and exercises. I understand that my journey in life is still long (as a privilege from God) and my future body is depending on me, I must not disappoint it.

Indeed, I have learned that menopause could be navigated with lifestyle adjustments and a positive mindset. This is not to discount the help provided to many women through HRT (Hormone Replacement Therapy).

As I finally transited to post-menopause, I reflected on the lessons learned and the strength gained throughout the process. It was a transformative experience that taught me resilience, self-compassion, and the importance of seeking knowledge and continuous learning.

In the end, the journey of menopause is not just about physical changes, but also about embracing a new chapter of life with grace, acceptance, understanding and compassion.

As I embraced this new chapter, I feel a deep calling to educate other women about menopause. Sharing the importance of understanding menopause as a natural part of the aging process, debunking misconceptions and cultural beliefs/myths that often surround it, particularlyin our African community.

I have seen firsthand that life does not end with menopause, rather it opens up new opportunities for intimacy, freedom from menstruation, renewed sense of purpose and personal growth.

Going forward, I envision a world where menopause education and support would be readily available to all women. I hope for a society where women would seek knowledge about menopause, overcome fears, and embrace this phase of life with confidence and grace.

Aging Is Not Dying!

Chapter 7

Some Beliefs And Myths Surrounding Menopause

Africa is home to diverse ethnic groups and cultures. As a result, attitudes, beliefs, and taboos related to menopause vary significantly from one culture to another. What is considered taboo in one community might be completely accepted in another. Even within a single country or region, you can find variations in how menopause is perceived which is influenced by beliefs of the people and existing myths. For example, urban areas may have different attitudes compared to rural regions.

These cultural factors profoundly influence how women experience menopause. For example, in cultures where menopause is celebrated, women may feel a sense of pride and positivity about this life stage. Conversely, in cultures where it is associated with secrecy or stigma, women may experience isolation, shame, trauma and vulnerability to being victims of schemers.

As societies modernise, attitudes toward menopause are also evolving. Urbanization, access to education/knowledge, and exposure to different worldviews through media can influence how women and their communities perceive menopause.

Here are some beliefs, myths and superstitions related to menopause in certain cultures in Africa:

1. Having sex with a menopausal woman will bring disease to the man:

This particular myth usually leads to marital challenges, isolation of the woman, leading sometimes to depression and also leading men in such cultures to become promiscuous or /and polygamists.

2. A man should not share the same room or bed with a menopausal woman:

This is similar to the above. The change in bedroom arrangements is one of the ways in which senior women are subtly told they are unfit for sexual encounters. This however, is incorrect and can be emotionally distressing for the woman.

3. Loss of fertility is a curse:

In some cultures, menopause is viewed as a woman's loss of fertility, and there can be superstitions or beliefs that associate it with curses or supernatural consequences of perceived actions in the past.

4. Menopause symptoms are spiritual:

Certain symptoms of menopause, like hot flashes or mood swings are attributed to supernatural causes or viewed as a woman being possessed by spirits in some communities.

5. Social stigma:

In some regions, women who have reached menopause may face social stigma or exclusion from certain activities or roles within the community due to beliefs about their diminished fertility or perceived changes in their status thereby limiting their social interactions.

6. Menopause should not be discussed openly:

In some cultures, discussing menopause openly is considered taboo. In such places, women may be reluctant to share their experiences thereby furthering misconceptions.

7. Menopause symptoms are caused by either, disease, witchcraft or sorcery:

Attributing the symptoms of menopause with witchcraft or sorcery especially, is what is responsible for some women seeking spiritual healing for their symptoms.

While there are beliefs or myths that negatively impact on the menopausal experience of women there are others that positively impact.

Some cultures see menopause as spiritually significant. Thus, the onset of menopause is with ceremonies conducted to mark this transition and also seek blessings for the woman's future. Such women are respected and considered wise elders due to their life experience and thus assume the role of a mentor and advisor within the family and community.

Again, it is essential to recognise that these beliefs and superstitions are not universally held across all African cultures, and views on menopause can vary widely. Moreover, as societies evolve and access to education and healthcare improve, many of these myths are being challenged and replaced by more informed perspectives on menopause.

In modern times, healthcare professionals, organisations and passionate individuals (like me) work to provide information and support for women going through this natural life stage.

It is important for the woman, having been exposed to such information to discover the beliefs and myths surrounding menopause in her culture and initiate conversation with her spouse for the purpose of enlightening him, and also collaborate with other women and understanding men to burst such beliefs and myths.

Aging Is Not Dying!

Chapter 8

Managing Menopause:

A Simple Guide To Symptoms Relief

Menopause is a natural phase of life that brings about various physical and emotional changes.

While these changes are part of getting older, they can sometimes cause discomfort and interrupt daily routines. Menopausal symptoms can be mild, moderate, or severe, and each woman's experience is unique.

Thankfully, menopause does not have to be a time of suffering. There are simple strategies and management options you can explore to manage symptoms, improve your quality of life, and embrace this new phase with confidence.

Before I give an overview of the options and strategies, I like to emphasize that, for me, the number one strategy is to stay informed through reputable sources, books, and online platforms.

Educating yourself about menopause will empower you to have informed discussions with your healthcare provider, ask relevant questions, and actively participate in decisions regarding your care.

Below is an overview of key management options you can explore to alleviate menopause symptoms and enhance your overall well-being. In the following chapters, each one shall receive a focus and further explanation.

1. Non-Hormonal Options

a. Lifestyle Modifications

-Healthy Eating

-Regular Exercise

-Stress Reduction Techniques

-Quality sleep

-Hormone-Friendly Lifestyle, which includes limiting alcohol or quitting altogether, quitting smoking, and maintaining a healthy weight.

It is important to note again that each person's experience with menopause is unique, and the impact of lifestyle factors may vary. Consulting with healthcare professionals, nutritionists, or fitness experts can provide personalized guidance based on your specific needs and health conditions.

b. Medications

Non-hormonal medications are often prescribed to manage various symptoms, including mood-related ones.

From experience and interaction with women, this option can turn a woman into a mobile pharmacy, especially when the root cause of her symptoms is not recognized as a sign of menopause. Nevertheless, it's important to relieve pain and discomfort, especially when they affect the quality of your day to day function.

c. Herbal supplements, natural remedies, and alternative therapies

Certain herbal supplements, acupuncture, or relaxation techniques have been used to alleviate menopause symptoms.

While some women find relief with herbal supplements or alternative practices, it's advised to consult with your healthcare provider before incorporating them into your regimen, especially with a view to ruling out dangerous drug interactions.

By exploring and implementing lifestyle modifications, you can alleviate menopause symptoms, enhance your overall well-being, and embrace this transformative phase of life with greater ease and vitality.

2. Hormone Replacement Therapy (HRT):

HRT involves replacing the hormones, such as estrogen and progesterone, that decline during menopause. This treatment aims to alleviate symptoms by restoring hormone levels.

HRT may be effective in managing menopause; however, it has potential risks. Therefore, it's important to have an open discussion with your healthcare provider about the benefits and potential risks, considering your individual health profile.

3. Regular health check-ups:

Maintaining regular health check-ups and screenings is essential during menopause. Stay in touch with your healthcare provider, gynecologist, or menopause specialist to monitor your overall health, discuss any concerns, and receive appropriate screenings or tests.

Personally, despite my knowledge and insight on this subject, I submit myself to an annual medical checkup, which always includes a mammogram. This I have done for nine years, and it has greatly helped me take responsibility for my well-being.

This has in no way reduced my faith in God

as my sustainer, but rather communicated to Him (I believe) that I am a faithful custodian of the body and life He has given me.

Let me chip this in for the benefit of everyone (men and women). We must not be careless with our health and go on neglecting principles for healthy living. If you recognize your body as the temple of God, keep it well to honor Him.

4. Mental Health Support:

If you are experiencing significant emotional challenges, such as mood swings, anxiety, or depression, consider seeking mental health support. Mental health professionals, such as psychologists or therapists, can help you navigate the emotional aspects of menopause and provide strategies to improve your well-being and overall quality of life.

I have added this here because I have encountered women with stories that touch the heart in their menopause journey and are a little messed up mentally.

5. Support groups and community:

Connecting with others who are going through similar experiences (offline or online) can provide a sense of validation and help you feel less alone during this transformative phase.

This can offer valuable insights, shared experiences, and emotional support.

In conclusion, remember that every woman's experience with menopause is unique, and it may take time to find the management options that work best for you. Be patient with yourself and stay open to trying different approaches.

It is also essential to consult with healthcare professionals for personalized guidance, especially if you have specific concerns or underlying medical conditions. They will assess your individual health profile, discuss your symptoms, and recommend the most suitable treatment options based on your needs and preferences.

Menopause is a chapter in your life story,

one that can be filled with wisdom, self-discovery, and renewed vitality.

Don't let menopause hold you back.

Take charge, stay cool, and get ready to thrive with "Managing Menopause."

Aging Is Not Dying!

Chapter 9

The Importance Of A Balanced Diet, Regular Exercise, And Adequate Sleep In Alleviating Menopause Symptoms

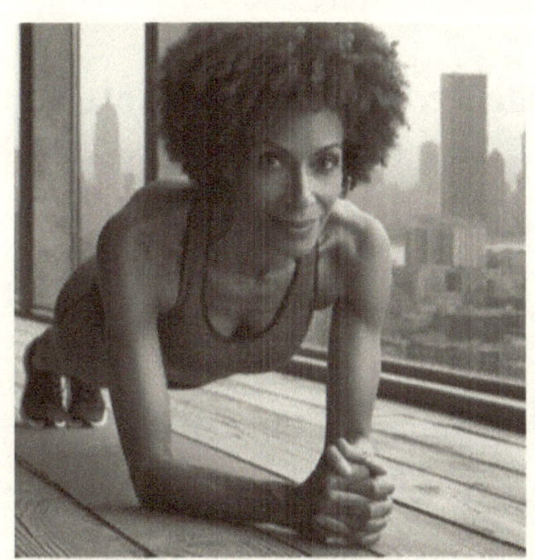

image created with Microsoft Bing AI Image Creator

Maintaining a healthy lifestyle is crucial

during menopause as it can significantly impact your physical and emotional well-being.

With the powerful trio of a balanced diet, regular exercise, and adequate sleep, you can navigate this natural transition with more ease and grace.

These simple yet powerful lifestyle changes can help alleviate symptoms, boost your overall health, and ensure that menopause becomes a manageable and, at times, even empowering experience

Let's explore each of them:

1. Balanced Diet:

A balanced diet is a powerful ally in alleviating the symptoms of menopause and promoting overall well-being.

Here's how:

- Hormone Balance: Nutrient-dense foods support hormonal balance. Foods rich in phytoestrogens, such as soy and flaxseeds, mimic the body's estrogen and can help alleviate hot flashes and mood swings.

- Weight Management: Menopause often brings unwanted weight gain. A balanced diet can help maintain a healthy weight, reducing the risk of obesity-related complications.

- Bone Health: Osteoporosis becomes a concern during menopause. Foods rich in calcium and vitamin D, like leafy greens, can help keep your bones strong.

- Heart Health: Cardiovascular health is crucial. Incorporating whole grains, fruits, and vegetables in your diet can help reduce the risk of heart disease. Over indulgence of consumption of processed food can trigger or aggravate symptoms.

- Hydration: Staying hydrated by drinking plenty of water is important for overall health and can help manage symptoms like dry skin and vaginal dryness.

2. Regular Exercise:

Engaging in regular physical activity offers numerous benefits during menopause.

Exercise may be the last thing on your mind when dealing with menopause symptoms, but it's a powerful tool:

- Mood Elevation: Exercise triggers the release of endorphins, which can help combat mood swings and depression.

- Weight Control: Regular physical activity boosts metabolism and helps control weight gain.

- Bone Strength: Weight-bearing exercises like walking and strength training can improve bone density.

- Adequate Sleep: Exercise can improve sleep quality and help with insomnia, a common menopausal complaint.

Aim for a combination of aerobic exercises,

such as brisk walking, swimming, or cycling, and strength training exercises to maintain muscle mass and bone density.

Consult with a healthcare professional or a fitness expert to determine the best exercise routine for your specific needs and capabilities.

3. Adequate Sleep:

Sleep is the body's reset button, and during menopause, it can be elusive making it difficult (for some women) to fall asleep or stay asleep as desired.

Here's why sleep is essential:

- Mood Stabilization: Adequate sleep helps regulate mood and reduce irritability.

- Energy Restoration: Menopause-related fatigue can be combated by getting enough sleep.

- Cognitive Function: Good sleep enhances memory, concentration, and overall brain function.

- Immune Support: A well-rested body can better fight off infections and illnesses.

It will benefit you to create a relaxing bedtime routine, maintain a comfortable sleep environment, and prioritize regular sleep patterns.

If menopause symptoms like night sweats or insomnia interfere with your sleep, consider using cooling bedding, wearing moisture-wicking sleepwear, or utilizing relaxation techniques to promote better rest.

In summary, by making healthy lifestyle choices, incorporating a balanced diet, regular exercise, and adequate sleep into your lifestyle, you can optimize your well-being during menopause and enjoy a smoother transition into this new phase of life.

Several benefits you can experience include:

- Reduced severity and frequency of hot flashes and night sweats.

- Improved mood and decreased risk of mood swings and irritability.

- Better management of weight and decreased risk of weight gain.

- Enhanced bone health and reduced risk of osteoporosis.

- Improved cardiovascular health and reduced risk of heart disease.

- Increased energy levels and overall vitality.

- Better stress management and improved emotional well-being.

It's important to note again that each person's experience with menopause is unique, and the impact of lifestyle factors may vary. What works for one might not work for another. It's essential to consult with your healthcare provider to create a personalized plan based on your specific needs and health conditions.

Embrace these lifestyle changes as opportunities for self-care and empowerment, and remember to listen to your body's cues, making adjustments as necessary along your menopause journey.

Aging Is Not Dying!

Chapter 10

Understanding the Available Medical Interventions: Hormone Replacement Therapy (HRT) and Non-Hormonal Options

When managing menopause symptoms, understanding the available medical interventions is crucial. Healthcare professionals can guide you through various treatment options, including both hormonal and non-hormonal approaches.

Let's explore these interventions:

1. Hormone Replacement Therapy (HRT):

HRT involves replacing the hormones, such as estrogen and progesterone, that decline during menopause. This treatment aims to alleviate symptoms by restoring hormone levels, that is, rebalancing the essential hormones involved in menopause.

There are different types of HRT available:

a. Estrogen Therapy: Estrogen-only therapy is prescribed for women who have had a hysterectomy {surgery to remove a woman's womb(uterus)}, as they do not need progesterone.

b. Combined hormone therapy, which includes both estrogen and progesterone. This is recommended for women with an intact uterus to protect the uterine lining.

Delivery Methods:

HRT can be administered through various methods, including oral tablets, patches, gels, creams, vaginal rings, or injections. Your healthcare provider will consider factors such as your symptoms, medical history, and personal preferences when recommending the most suitable delivery method for you.

Benefits and Risks:

HRT is effective in managing menopause symptoms such as hot flashes, night sweats, vaginal dryness, and mood swings. It can also help prevent osteoporosis. However, HRT (according to available medical information), may have potential risks, including an increased risk of blood clots, stroke, breast cancer, and cardiovascular issues.

It's important to have an open discussion with your healthcare provider about the benefits and potential risks associated with HRT, considering your individual health profile.

2. Non-Hormonal Options:

If HRT is not suitable for you or you prefer non-hormonal interventions, there are several alternatives available:

a. Medications: Non-hormonal medications, are often prescribed to manage hot flashes and mood-related symptoms. These medications work by affecting brain chemicals that regulate body temperature and mood.

b. Herbal Supplements: Certain herbal supplements, have been used to alleviate menopause symptoms.

While some women find relief with these supplements, their effectiveness varies.

It's crucial to seek guidance from your healthcare provider, particularly if you are already taking prescribed medications for other health conditions, before integrating these remedies into yourroutine.

c. Vaginal Estrogen Therapy: For women experiencing vaginal dryness, discomfort, or urinary symptoms, vaginal estrogen therapy may be recommended. This involves applying a small amount of estrogen cream, tablet, or ring directly to the vagina to relieve symptoms locally.

An open communication with your healthcare provider will ensure you make informed decisions about your treatment plan, maximizing the benefits while minimizing potential risks.

In addition, regular follow-up appointments will allow them to monitor your progress, adjust treatment if necessary, and address any concerns or questions you may have.

In conclusion, it is my firm recommendation to initially embrace lifestyle modifications as your primary approach to manage menopause symptoms. Reserve the consideration of medical interventions for instances where your symptoms remain unrelieved, causing prolonged discomfort, or significantly interfering with your daily life.

Aging Is Not Dying!

Chapter 11

A Positive Outlook

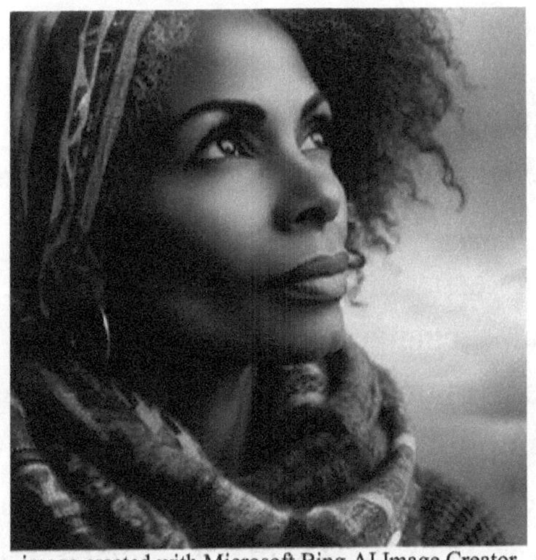
image created with Microsoft Bing AI Image Creator

Staying positive and empowering yourself to make informed choices for your health and well-being during menopause.

A positive outlook during menopause is crucial, as it empowers women to make informed choices about their health and well-being. In addition, it helps women navigate this transformative phase with confidence and make decisions that align with their needs and preferences.

Here are some ways to ensure a positive outlook and empower yourself during menopause:

1. Get Informed

Equip yourself with accurate and comprehensive information about menopause to make informed choices. This should cover various aspects of menopause, including physical changes, emotional well-being, treatment options, and lifestyle modifications. By equipping yourself with knowledge, you not only eliminate fear and panic, you also empower yourself to make choices for your well-being based on a clear understanding.

2. Locate a Supportive Community

Connect with other women going through menopause, share experiences, and offer encouragement to one another. In such community (online or offline), you can find solace, validation, and guidance.

Peer support do play a significant role in promoting a positive outlook and empowering women to take charge of their health.

3. Use of Positive Language

Speak positively when discussing menopause to shift the narrative from decline to empowerment. Focus on the opportunities for growth, self-discovery, and renewed vitality that menopause brings. Celebrate the resilience and wisdom that women gain during this phase of life. By reframing the conversation, you can foster a positive outlook and empower yourself to embrace the changes with optimism.

4. Prioritize Self-Care

Take care of your well-being by engaging in activities that promote physical, emotional, and mental health.

Seek resources and guidance on self-care practices such as exercise, healthy eating, mindfulness, stress management, and relaxation techniques. Doing this will empower you to navigate menopause with resilience and vitality.

5. Personal Approach

I can't help but remind you again that each woman's experience with menopause is unique. While some breeze through menopause, some face some difficult symptoms. Embrace your own individual journey and make choices that align with your specific needs and preferences. Be open to consulting with healthcare professionals, therapists, or specialists who can provide personalized guidance based on your unique circumstance. Doing this will enable you to make decisions that support your overall well-being.

6. Holistic Well-being

You can adopt a holistic approach to your well-being during menopause. Be open to address the physical, emotional, and mental aspects of your health.

It's important to pay attention to nurturing

relationships at this time, maintain a healthy lifestyle, practice self-compassion, and seek support when needed. Again, by considering the whole person, you empower yourself to make informed choices that promote your overall well-being during menopause.

Having a positive outlook and empowering yourself during menopause is a process. You will need to continuously seek resources, support, and encouragement to ensure you are empowered to make informed choices.

Remember, Menopause is not a decline, but rather a chance to embrace a new chapter of life with wisdom, vitality, and a deeper understanding of yourself.

I urge you to embrace the opportunities that menopause presents and seize the chance to create a fulfilling and empowered life during and after this transformative phase.

Aging Is Not Dying!

Chapter 12

A Summary of Lifestyle Modifications for Embracing Menopause with Confidence and Grace

As your body undergoes changes, so can your lifestyle. Here are some practical and empowering lifestyle modifications to navigate this phase with grace and vitality:

1. Healthy Nutrition:

   - Prioritize a well-balanced diet rich in fruits, vegetables, whole grains, and lean proteins.

   - Include calcium-rich foods to support bone health, as women are more susceptible to bone density loss during menopause.

- Stay hydrated. Water is not just a beverage; it's a vital companion in this journey.

2. Regular Exercise:

- Engage in regular physical activity, including both aerobic exercises and strength training.

- Exercise helps manage weight, boosts mood, and contributes to overall well-being.

- Find activities you enjoy, whether it's dancing, or walking, and make them a regular part of your routine.

3. Quality Sleep:

- Prioritize good sleep hygiene. Create a relaxing bedtime routine and ensure your sleep environment is conducive to rest.

- Adequate sleep is crucial for mood regulation, cognitive function, and overall health.

4. Stress Management:

   - Explore stress-reducing practices like meditation or deep breathing.

   - Consider activities that bring joy and relaxation, such as reading, gardening, or spending time in nature.

5. Social Connection:

   - Nurture social relationships. Share your experiences with friends or join support groups.

   - Connection and shared experiences can provide emotional support during thistransformative time.

6. Hormone-Friendly Habits:

   - Limit caffeine and alcohol intake, as they can impact sleep and worsen symptoms.

- Quit smoking if applicable. Smoking can intensify hot flashes and increase the risk of osteoporosis.

7. Wardrobe Adjustments:

Hot flashes is one of the common symptoms of menopause, for this;

- Embrace comfortable clothing, Choose breathable fabrics and layers for easy temperature control.

- Invest in good-quality sleepwear for a more restful night.

8. Regular Health Check-ups:

- Schedule regular check-ups with your healthcare provider.

- Discuss symptoms, concerns, and any necessary screenings or preventive measures.

9. Holistic Approaches:

- Explore holistic therapies like herbal supplements, or aromatherapy for symptom relief.

- Consult with healthcare professionals to ensure safety and effectiveness.

Menopause is a new beginning. By embracing these lifestyle modifications, you empower yourself to navigate this phase with resilience, embracing the wisdom and beauty that comes with the journey.

I wish you a vibrant and fulfilling menopausal chapter in your life!

Aging Is Not Dying!

Chapter 13

Nurturing Relationships and Sexual Health in Menopause

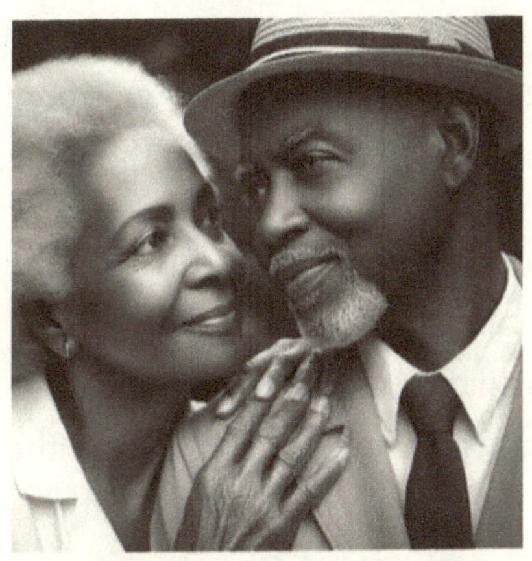

image created with Microsoft Bing AI Image Creator

Menopause can significantly impact relationships, touching on various aspects, including emotional, physical, and sexual dimensions. However, with this awareness, I call on women to change the narrative by preparing for this transformative phase of life and be ready to respond to it positively and have the best time of their relationship and sexual intimacy with their partner.

Emotional Changes

Hormonal fluctuations during menopause can lead to mood swings, irritability, and emotional sensitivity.

All these symptoms, coupled with the challenges of this life phase, can contribute to increased stress and anxiety in the woman.

These changes might affect how women communicate and interact with their partners, thus, partners are encouraged to provide additional emotional support during this time.

Physical Challenges

Menopause can bring about physical changes, such as weight gain or changes in skin and hair. These alterations may impact self-esteem and, consequently, intimate relationships.

In addition, symptoms like hot flashes and night sweats can disrupt sleep, leading to fatigue during the day.

Partners should be understanding and supportive of changes in energy levels.

Sexual Changes

Fluctuations in hormone levels can contribute to a decrease in libido and vaginal dryness. The former might affect the frequency of sexual activity in a relationship, while the latter can make it uncomfortable or painful for the woman.

While sexual dynamics might shift, maintaining intimacy through non-sexual means, such as affection and emotional connection, becomes vital. In addition, open communication with partner and exploring solutions like lubricants can be essential.

Communication Challenges

Mood swings and emotional changes may lead to misunderstandings if not communicated effectively. This is because sometimes, a partner might not fully grasp the physical and emotional challenges of menopause. Understanding, education and open conversations are therefore crucial.

Children Leaving Home

Menopause can coincide with the children leaving home (empty nest syndrome).

This is another major shift for a woman already going through menopause and can contribute to emotional changes leading to a shift in roles and relationship dynamics, Couples are expected to adapt to a new phase of life together. However, if the relationship had not been carefully nurtured before now, difficulty may arise.

In essence, the key to navigating the impact of menopause on relationships lies in open communication, empathy, and a willingness to adapt to the changes that this transformative phase brings. Couples who approach menopause as a shared journey can strengthen their relationship through mutual support and understanding.

Tips For Couples To Maintain Intimacy During and After Menopause

1. Open Communication

Openly communicate about the physical and emotional changes each partner may be experiencing. Express your feelings, concerns, and desires regarding intimacy.

2. Educate Yourselves

Take the time to educate yourselves about the effects of menopause on sexual health. Consider reading books or articles together to understand each other's perspectives.

3. Explore Non-Sexual Intimacy

Strengthen emotional bonds through activities that promote understanding and closeness. Spend quality time together doing things you both enjoy.

4. Experiment with New Activities

Discover new hobbies or activities you can enjoy together. You can consider planning trips or experiences that can create shared memories.

5. Prioritize Emotional Intimacy

Discuss your hopes, dreams, and aspirations. Allow yourselves to be vulnerable with each other, sharing both joys and concerns.

6. Sensual Touch

Engage in non-sexual touch, such as cuddling, holding hands, or gentle massages. Explore each other's bodies without the pressure of sexual expectations.

7. Laugh Together

Share lighthearted moments and find humor in daily life. Keep a sense of playfulness in your relationship.

8. Prioritize Self-Care

Focus on your individual well-being, including physical and mental health. Support each other in self-care practices that contribute to overall well-being.

9. Professional Guidance

Consider couples counseling or therapy to address any challenges and enhance communication. Seek professional guidance on maintaining a satisfying intimate life.

10. Adapt and Innovate

Be open to trying new things in the bedroom. Explore different ways to connect intimately that is comfortable for both of you.

11. Create a Romantic Environment

Schedule regular date nights to focus on each other. Surprise each other with small, thoughtful gestures to maintain a sense of romance.

12. Celebrate Milestones

Celebrate anniversaries and other relationship milestones. Also, acknowledge and celebrate each other's personal achievements.

Remember, maintaining intimacy is a shared responsibility that requires understanding, patience, and adaptability. Embrace the changes together, stay connected emotionally, and find new ways to nurture your relationship.

Breaking Stereotypes: Menopausal Women Redefining Love and Romance

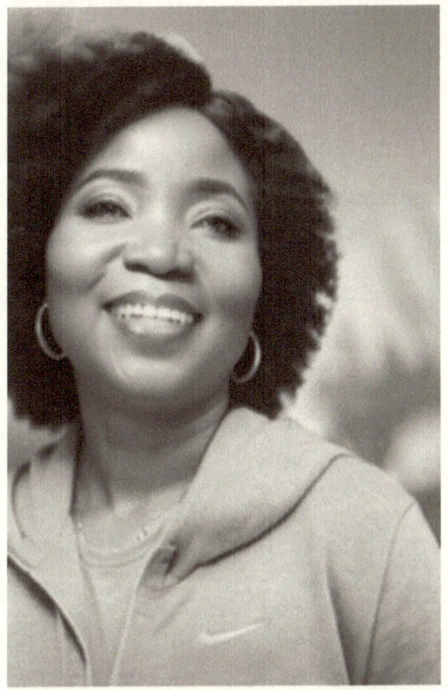

'Denike Owolabi (image enhanced with Remini AI Image Enhancer)

As I strolled down my Facebook feed, a post interrupted my usual scroll. It was the honest post of a woman in the revered club of menopause, though single (life happened).

She narrated how she suddenly found herself on the receiving end of attention and affection from younger men, all asking her out and eager to get into serious relationships. Interesting!

The comments section became a drama arena, but the digital drama kind. Some were tossing metaphorical roses, cheering her on for daring to embrace love and romance during the menopausal season of life. Meanwhile, others, equipped with their keyboards as swords, questioned the authenticity of her newfound romance or her capability to embrace love.

Amidst this uproar, one comment stood out like a neon sign in the dark.

This particular lady – let me call her the 'headmistress of love' – expressed surprise, shock, sheer disbelief really, that women in menopause would dare divert their attention from attending August meetings and conducting grandmotherly activities like "omugwo" to entertaining thoughts of love and romance.

The audacity!

Is she for real? Ha ha ha! Her Surprise surprised me. It caught me off guard really. I mean, who says that menopause comes with an unwritten rulebook dictating a mandatory retirement of one's heart.

Come close!

Menopause isn't a declaration of "Goodbye Romance!" It's more of a "Hello, New Chapter". The idea that menopause should be a romance barrier is as outdated as my attempt at gymnastics in my secondary school days, it's bad.

Let me tell you – women in menopause are still the CEOs of love and affection. We are talking about smooches, hand-holding, hugs, sweet whispers and even some spicy bedroom intimacy that defy societal norms faster than you can say, "But, aren't they supposed to be engaged in omugwo somewhere?"

And here's the thing – menopause does not play musical chairs with dreams. No! Women in menopause can still chase their passions, rock the runway of life, and even have a worthy interest in beauty and fashion.

Menopause isn't a time to collect dust; it's a VIP pass to empowerment and self-discovery.

Move over stereotypes; the menopausal ladies are in town, and they aren't just here for "Omugwo"!

See, women in menopause are proving that love and all that accompany it aren't just for the younger generation. Take note!

Love, my friends, is ageless. Menopause is not a 'Restricted' section of the romance library. Love, for a menopausal woman can be spicy as the hottest pepper in the garden, no matter the age on the calendar.

That surprising comment, by the "Headmistress Of Love", my dear, highlights the need to break free from stereotypes and challenge the 'you-are-too-old-for-this' brigade.

What I am saying is, love and romance are not reserved for the Gen Z; they are universal experiences, available for all, no matter the season of life.

I really love that woman who shared her

experience. Her story threw a blow at societal norms and shattered stereotypes like a broken glass mirror, and stood up for women in menopause everywhere. She deserves a medal.

Hey woman! Think of menopause as the opening of a new chapter filled with possibilities fornew adventures, getting to know yourself better, personal growth, and the possibility of some awesome continuation, or start of love stories.

Cheers to that!

As I close, let's remember – love, like a good wine, gets better with age.

Cheers to the women in menopause, still rocking the stage and proving that love knows no boundaries, no matter how many candles are on the birthday cake.

Aging Is Not Dying!

Omugwo is a tradition rooted in the South Eastern part of Nigeria, where an older woman provides care and support to a new mother and her newborn. It's a beautiful practice centered around nurturing and assistance during the early days of motherhood.

Aging Is Not Dying!

Chapter 14

Concluding Thought: Embracing the Power of Menopause

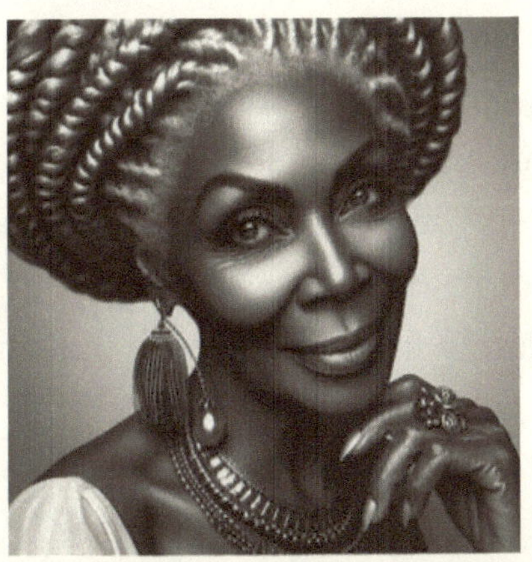

image created with Microsoft Bing AI Image Creator

Remember, dear reader, that menopause is not an ending, but a beginning - a gateway to a new chapter of life filled with personal growth, self-discovery, and renewed vitality. It is a time to honor our bodies, cherish our experiences, and embrace the incredible power that resides within us.

As African women, we have a rich heritage of resilience, strength, and wisdom passed down through generations. Let us honor that legacy by embracing menopause as a transformative phase, weaving our stories into the fabric of our culture, and empowering future generations of women.

So, as we bid farewell to these pages, let us carry the knowledge, insights, and inspiration gained throughout this journey. Let us continue to uplift one another, challenge societal norms, and advocate for the well-being of African women during this profound life transition.

Embrace your power

Embrace the beauty, the resilience, and the profound wisdom that menopause has bestowed upon you.

Embrace the possibilities that lie ahead and

create a future filled with joy, purpose, and fulfillment.

Embrace the menopause phase of your life, and let your light shine brightly, inspiring others to embark on their own journeys of self-empowerment and growth.

Aging Is Not Dying!

With love,

'Denike Owolabi